The Lost Years

By S. M. Jones

The Lost Years
Copyright ©2018 by SM Jones
All rights reserved. Printed in the United States of America.

No part of this book may be used or reproduced in any manner whatsoever without the express written permission of the author.

The following is a true-life account of the author's own experiences and from the author's own perspective.

Published by CLC Publishing, LLC, Yukon, OK.

ISBN: 978-1721762842

Non-Fiction/Mental Health/Alzheimer's

"To focus on something you want to achieve – no matter how small – is more relevant than focusing on something you've already achieved." – SM Jones

Preface

Lost = missing, gone, vanished, nowhere to be found

Years = existence, being, living, time

When speaking of a loved one afflicted with the dreaded disease named Alzheimer's, what words do you think of?

What is lost? Everything. Once it's gone, it's gone. Never to be attained, remembered or felt.

Our memories are our life, our being. It's the birthday party many years ago, the surprise wedding anniversary celebration and the vacation trip of a lifetime.

But when the memory is gone, it's as if none of that ever happened. We remember. The afflicted don't.

When the memory of your loved one has been lost, and you and what you were to that person is the lost memory, what happens then? When you are the object of that lost memory, it is as if you cease to exist to that person—as if you were never born. You just become a 'nice' person who visits them with trinkets, smiles, many hugs, and an unseen broken heart.

This story is dedicated to the memory of my mother, Marie. A memory that she lost far too long before she lost her fight for life.

1

The sound of the phone in the background gave me a well-deserved break as we finalized counting the late RSVPs for our daughter's wedding. In approximately three weeks, we would throw the biggest party of our lives. The past eleven months of planning this wedding had gone effortlessly; sixteen people in the wedding party, the reception to be held where we wanted, and 100 confirmed guests.

To me, two of the most important guests would be flying in from Florida; my parents. I couldn't wait to see them as it had been almost two years since the last visit.

"Hello?" I answered, taking in a deep breath as if a sign of obtaining a relaxing moment.

"Honey, it's Mom." I recognized the familiar, 'don't worry' tone at the very first word.

"What's wrong?" I questioned, noting severe hesitation in my own voice.

"There's nothing to worry about, but your father is in the hospital. Don't get upset, it's just some bad stomach bug. We'll be at the wedding, so don't worry."

With things perfect up 'til now, we finished the call with that 'oh no' feeling in the pit of my stomach. I was hopeful that the smooth sailing would continue, as my father's timing was always a bit off center. This is actually something that I could have predicted.

My phone call to Dad after dinner was for the sole purpose of hearing his voice and to reassure my positive thinking. His response was what I expected. He had already informed the nurses that he had to be out of the hospital in a week. His airline tickets were purchased, and he was flying to Pennsylvania for his granddaughter's wedding.

I spoke with him daily, and Mom too, but I soon learned some disturbing news. Despite finding out that Dad was now hooked up to some tubes, he still insisted that he was fine and would still be there in time for the wedding. After all, we still had about two weeks to go.

It was Saturday and we had just come back from shopping. The bags dropped from our arms onto the sofa and I plopped onto the overstuffed chair which seemed to call to me.

"I'm beat. Tomorrow is Mother's Day and our anniversary, and I'm going to sit around and do absolutely nothing," I swore, exhaling forcefully.

"You deserve it. You've been running around like crazy to make sure everything is perfect for the wedding. All the plans are finished, and you've done it. Tomorrow will be ours." My husband always put my needs first.

I noticed that the phone was blinking. 'One message' glowed in crimson red. I smiled as I walked towards the phone, not knowing this would be the last time I would smile for the next seven days.

"This message is for Susan Smith. This is Venice Hospital. Please call when you receive this message."

I heard nothing after that, my heart sank. I felt sick to my stomach. My eyes never left the message machine. Noting the terrified look on my face, my husband handed me a pen and a tablet of paper and I called the number after I listened to the message for the second time.

The hospital operator's question blind-sided me when I asked to be connected to my father's room.

"Who's calling please?" Her voice was noticeably quieter. "This is Susan Smith, his daughter," my shaky voice trailed off at the end. "Just a moment, I'll connect you to the nurse's station." The phone went quiet, no comforting music, just dead silence.

"Mrs. Smith?" "Yes, I received a call and was put through to you instead of my father's room. What's wrong?"

"Mrs. Smith, I regret to inform you that your father passed away this evening." The words echoed in my head, banging back and forth between my ears like a bell ringing high noon.

No words needed to be said. The truth was known as my eyes filled with tears and at that point, anyone could have looked right through me.

I had learned that my father had finally gone home, and I called mom, tissues in hand. Mom's voice was subdued. She had been crying but was somewhat settled at this point. I felt terrible, being the only child, that I was a thousand miles away in Pennsylvania. I wanted to reach through the phone and hold her.

She had been with him, told him she was going to the cafeteria and returned about one-half hour later. On the way back to his room, she passed the Chapel and said she felt an unexplainable cool chill. Not seeing any open doors, she continued walking back to his room only to find it full of nurses, technicians, doctors, and large cumbersome, portable equipment.

For some reason, my father had gotten out of bed and was walking towards the chair to sit down. It appeared that a massive heart attack took his life immediately. There was nothing that could be done.

I called my daughter's fiancé and asked him to bring her home after I told him what had happened. I found out later that he didn't tell her until they were on our front steps and about to walk in the house. I called my son and told him to stay at his friend's house and that I would be in touch.

Our daughter withdrew temporarily. The weight of her grandfather's death, mixed with the excitement of her wedding in two weeks, was a lot for a young woman to consume all at once. I made flight arrangements for the next morning. I would leave at 8 AM; not soon enough for me. I called Mom, told her arrangements had been made and to expect me around 11 AM.

Before I knew it, I was in flight, on my anniversary, on Mother's Day, and on my way to see my mother, and say goodbye to my father.

Time passed so quickly. The plane landed, and her house was in view. I don't even remember the ride or the baggage checkout. I called the hospital and requested to visit with my father. He was going to be cremated and I wanted and needed to see him in the flesh before that happened. Two years had been too long for not seeing him.

Within a week, a church service was performed which included a Masonic Funeral with Military honors. The last thing I remember was hearing "Taps" and being handed a folded American Flag and a brass box displaying the praying hands on the side. I was holding my father. It just didn't seem right.

We emptied Mom's refrigerator and two days later her and I flew back to Pennsylvania, along with several of her suitcases, as we had made arrangements that she would spend the rest of the summer with us. Seven days to go and all the wedding plans were complete. Everything was in order and to my surprise, Mom was doing very well.

We arrived at the church with more than enough time to relax. As my son-in-law-to-be was a volunteer with the local fire company, a fireman's wedding theme was in place and many of those in attendance wore uniforms. Black bands had been affixed to the badges since it was still within the 30-day mourning period for a fallen fire-fighter; my father had also been a member of the same fire company and an honorary active member. I had temporarily forgotten, and the black bands brought tears to my eyes. My makeup had to be reapplied.

The beautiful wedding ceremony on a sunlit afternoon only brought more tears. Joy and sadness both rested on my heart for the remainder of the day.

The reception was joyful, and Mom spent a lot of time reflecting with my mother-in-law who had also become a widow two years earlier. Ironically, both their husbands passed within a few days of each other, all around Mother's Day and my anniversary. These dates would remain in my mind forever.

2

Mom spent the rest of the summer with us. I tried to keep her as busy as I could. I signed her up at the Senior Center where she went every morning and gave her the opportunity to spend time with others her age. With me working during the week, I thought this would help keep her busy. On the weekends, I would take her to visit areas of interest always thinking that if I kept her mind busy, she wouldn't constantly be talking about daddy; but she did. We visited many places she'd never seen when she lived here and took her to visit many old friends that she hadn't seen since moving to Florida about ten years ago.

The wedding had been in early June and now it was early October. The temperature was beginning to cool down and she was ready to go home, back to warmer weather. To be honest, we needed a little time of our own too, but we enjoyed the time we had with her.

We said goodbye at the airport, we cried again, and she headed home.

The newlyweds were gone living at their place, and my home was back to normal. With the exception of missing my father dearly, I was looking forward to some desperately needed rest and some normalcy back in my life. Unfortunately, that feeling was short lived.

Two weeks after Mom returned home, she called me at work one day. I questioned her surprise phone call.

"Hi, Mom. Good to hear from you. What's up?" I spoke quickly trying to get her off the work phone so I could call her tonight from home.

"I was just thinking about you and wanted to give you a call." She answered with an upbeat voice that soon took an awkward turn.

"I was thinking of coming up for a visit. I haven't seen you in a while." Her statement strangled my mind. The phone almost fell from my hand. She had just spent over four months with us and had only left two weeks ago. Yet, she's saying she hasn't seen us in a while. The confrontation within me immediately spoke up.

"Mom, you just left us two weeks ago after being here for over four months!" I responded trying not to be too forceful with my statement.

"What?" Her quiet voice responded, ending in a confused but obvious whisper.

"Mom, you were here for Dawn's wedding after daddy died, remember? It was in late May and then you stayed the entire summer with us. You left two weeks ago, and I've spoken with you about every other day since you returned home."

The silence was deafening on the other end of the phone and the thought of this conversation was eating me up inside. What was going on?

"I don't remember." She paused. "I remember daddy dying and the wedding a while ago, but I thought I hadn't seen you in some time."

I assured her that it was probably still hard on her, especially with just returning to the house since his death, and suggested that she join the singles club and keep busy with the other widows and widowers at the clubhouse in her development. One of the couples there actually grew up with her and Dad in Philadelphia, and I suggested that she contact them to assist in keeping her busy. I thought that would help.

Unfortunately, it didn't. The next two months were disastrous. I never had a chance to call daily, which is what my plan was; she was calling me. Her phone calls didn't bother me, I loved speaking with her, but the subjects of our conversations were beginning to worry me more and more with every call.

The same subjects, the same tidbits, night after night, after night. When I couldn't keep it in anymore, I sat down with my husband. I had a terrified look on my face and a heavy heart.

"Something's definitely wrong with Mom" I whispered, the words barely escaping my lips falling off at the end.

"What's the matter? What's wrong?"

"Our conversations were the same over and over again. She keeps repeating everything. Every phone call is practically the duplication of the one the day before. I'm afraid to even think it, but she is showing all the signs of Alzheimer's or dementia. I don't know the difference, but I'm going to start to research it. She's so far away and there's no family with her. I have to understand what's going on."

He didn't have an answer. I don't think he really understood what we were about to head into, and neither did I nor my family.

It was the middle of November and I received a very disturbing phone call one night shortly after dinner.

"Hello?" I answered on an upbeat note as I was wrapping some early Christmas presents.

"Is this Susan?" An unknown upset voice asked.

"Yes, who's this?"

"Susan, this is Mrs. Anderson from your mother's development. I really hate making this phone call, but we have to discuss your mother."

Before she could continue, my emotions took over the phone call.

"What's wrong with my mother? I just spoke with her about an hour ago."

"Please don't get me wrong Susan; your mother needs some help." Her voice was hesitant but firm. A tone I immediately realized; one that I did not like.

"What do you mean, help?"

"Susan, your mother is getting confused, very confused and I hate to say it, but she is beginning to constantly bother some of her neighbors." Her voice ended quickly.

Our conversation continued in a direction that was unknown to me and one that I did not like. Apparently, Mom had been calling her friends and would ask them to drive her to the food store or to the singles' meetings. She hadn't renewed her drivers' license when she moved to Florida. Her friends would call her to let her know what time they would pick her up and she would tell them she didn't want to go or ask why they were calling her.

Half an hour later, she'd call them back and leave a message or talk to them and would say she'd want to go to the store or somewhere. It appears that this had been going on since Mom returned home in October.

I assured Mrs. Anderson that I would talk with Mom tomorrow, and hopefully get her on the right path. Mrs. Anderson, however, was not on the same line of communication with me. Her last statement basically stated that if there was no change in Mom's habit, then she would be back on the phone with me again, without delay.

I hung up the phone, with my husband noticing the obviously distressed look on my face.

I explained the situation and the repetitive pattern that Mom had fallen into.

"She is starting to forget everything. Our telephone calls are constant reminders. She doesn't remember anything within a short time frame, but she has no problem remembering anything that happened a long time ago. I'll talk to her and see what's going on."

I walked into the kitchen, made myself some coffee because I knew this was not going to be a good night after all.

One hour and one coffee pot later, I walked back into the living room and looked around with a blank stare.

"How bad is it?" He wanted to know the truth and he needed to know how bad the situation really was.

"It's bad. She says she doesn't even remember calling her neighbors to go anywhere. She says they call her and ask her. She says she doesn't want to go to the singles' group as she misses daddy too much. She still says she hasn't seen us in over a year, but she does remember the wedding. Telling her to stop bothering the neighbors isn't doing any good if she doesn't remember calling them in the first place." I hesitated and was afraid to speak what my mind was thinking. "I think we have the beginning of a serious problem."

I put the wrapping paper away with the unwrapped presents and got ready for bed, wanting to put my brain to sleep for the night.

Thanksgiving came and went. She said she had a nice turkey dinner up at the clubhouse and we entered into December on what I felt was a quiet note. Unfortunately, that quiet note wasn't long enough.

3

It was the first week in December and Mrs. Anderson's uninvited phone call ruined a Christmas shopping night out. We were walking out the door when the phone rang, and I recognized the Florida area code immediately; but not the phone number.

"I have to get this call, it's not from Mom." I hesitated with my eyes fixed on the number. My mouth was dry and it was very difficult to answer.

"Hello."

"Susan, this is Mrs. Anderson, again." The shaky, but firm, elderly voice stammered on the other end of the line a thousand miles away.

"Yes, Mrs. Anderson, what can I do for you this evening?" I answered her not really wanting to hear anything she had to say.

"It's your mother, again. It's the same as before, only it's getting worse. I'm sorry to say but you have to do something with your mother."

The words went through my heart like a blazing hot knife. Mom was worse, calling everyone, giving them a hard time and was very confused. Her final remark made the reality of the issue very clear.

"Susan, we don't care what you do, but she is your responsibility, not ours. We hate telling you this, but it's the truth and hope that you can address this problem by the end of the year. You need to take responsibility for your mother. We cannot."

I was furious, hurt and angered. She just called my mother a problem. How dare she? I responded with the feelings that were now raging inside me.

"Don't worry, Mrs. Anderson! You won't have the problem to deal with after New Year's." With that, I slammed the phone down so hard it fell to the floor.

I tried to compose myself. I knew we had to talk, I just didn't know how to start the conversation.

"What's wrong now?" He searched for an answer, having an idea.

"After we do some shopping we'll stop for coffee and discuss it; not now."

I surprised myself on being able to concentrate on shopping at this point, but I did pretty well finding some fantastic Christmas sales. By the time we stopped for coffee I had settled down to my normal self and spoke frankly with my husband.

I don't know how many cups of coffee I had, as every time the waiter went by I asked him to top off the cup. An uneaten piece of pie lay in front of me, only picked apart by my fork. I was an only child. The only one able to do anything with my mother, and something had to be done. By the end of our conversation, he had earned his wings in heaven. He had agreed to allow Mom to move in with us. She would use the bedroom I was planning on making a sitting room. The plans were made. I would take vacation the week between Christmas and New Years and we would go to Florida, pack her up and move her back to Pennsylvania with us.

We actually arrived on December 23, put together her artificial Christmas tree and celebrated Christmas like we hadn't done in a long time.

We rented the largest U-Haul we could, and the nightmare began with the packing. Mom and Dad had both been hoarders being raised by parents who dealt with the depression. The collections of butter tubs, newspapers and newspaper plastic bags proved that fact.

A folder belonging to my father caught not only my eye but my heart as well. As I read the words in front of me, I could do nothing but blink back tears. It was proof that Mom had been seeing a doctor, apparently under Dad's request, and his findings only topped off the thoughts hidden deep in my mind. **Mild Alzheimer's/Dementia, proven.** I read the report which was over a year old. They knew there was an issue, or at least Dad knew there was an issue, but never said a word to me. Whether he told Mom or not, I'll never know. I re-read the report several times to make sure I didn't miss anything.

Piece after piece of furniture was loaded into the van and then I dealt with the rest of the things. Dad's clothes were donated to the Goodwill and Mom decided to give a lot of things away to her friends in the park. The van couldn't hold one more item and the car was packed to the roof.

By December 29, we were in the car headed to Pennsylvania after she said goodbye to all her 'so-called' friends who were all in attendance to 'wish her well'. Several came to me to talk, but I excused myself not wanting to confront them at this point or at any other time.

The words I had previously read kept sounding in my mind. I wondered how bad it was and how bad it would get. But the biggest question was how long I would have her. I didn't know that much about the disease, but I did know that it took the soul of a person and their mind before actually taking their life. The thought that someday she would look at me and not know who I was, her only child, had already begun to eat at my insides.

My house never looked so good and neither did my kids. We rested for the next 24 hours, which included New Year's Eve, then began the work again. Her personal items were brought into our house and the remainder of her items went into storage.

The first thing I did was sign her back up at the Senior Center to return to the few friends she had made during the summer months. The only problem was she never remembered being there, so it was all new to her and she enjoyed herself very much. Life in our house was beginning very smoothly. Unfortunately, it wouldn't last as long as I had hoped and prayed.

Before we knew it, spring had flown by and summer was upon us. I'm sure the hot weather reminded Mom of Florida, but we didn't mention it too much because, believe it or not, she had only received one birthday card from one of her 'friends' that she left in the development. Other than that, she had not heard from anyone. I felt sorry for her. Thankfully, she had already forgotten many of the people that she had left.

My husband came home from work before me and met me in the driveway before going into the house.

"We are beginning to have a problem." he said, wiping his forehead in the 99-degree heat.

"Can't we discuss this in the air conditioning? It's stifling out here," I asked heading towards the door.

"Well, I guess if the house has cooled down by now."

I glanced at the condenser running normally on the side of the house. "Why wouldn't the house be cool? The air conditioner is running."

Just about this time, our neighbor came over to assist with the story. He had come over to thank us for helping to cool down the neighborhood. Not understanding what he was saying, I soon learned that for the past three hours, all of our windows were wide open, and the air conditioning was blowing out onto the street.

Mom had returned from the Center and feeling the hot temperatures outside, proceeded to open all the windows in the house, as my electric bill raced towards the clouds.

Mom couldn't understand why anyone would be shutting all the windows and stopping the warm air from coming in the house. She couldn't understand or remember that the air conditioner was running full force. I discussed it with her and thought she understood, but within the next couple weeks, the same happened again, more than once.

This upset Mom, as she couldn't remember our conversations and said she didn't even remember opening the windows. I was glad when the weather began to cool because the air conditioner was off and if she opened the windows, it was a welcomed breeze.

The next several seasons seemed to drag by and the atmosphere in my house was slowly changing. Mom was getting more and more confused and the tension in the home became thicker and thicker. We began having problems finding things as Mom, thinking that she was helping, would put things away or move things and finding them was not an interesting game.

If we went out, I would always call her on the phone to check in on her and thankfully she'd always answer; until one night.

"We have to go home, there's no answer on the phone." The panic in my voice elevated.

I ran up the front steps to find her contented watching TV and smiling like a little child, contented to be where she was.

"Hi, have a good time?" She asked upbeat and perky.

"Uh, yes, I just wanted to check on you since you didn't answer the phone when I called."

It was determined that she had heard the phone ringing, several times, but didn't know where it was to answer it.

Nothing had changed; the phone was where it always was. She just forgot its location.

4

The next couple of years played out the same pattern. Forgetting this and misplacing that. Even to her, it was becoming more and more obvious. She'd ask what was wrong and I'd blow the answer or even the conversation off, not wanting to tell her the ultimate demise.

One day, she put the question out to me and I felt awkward but compelled to tell her the truth. "Susan, what's wrong with me? Why can't I remember anything and why am I so confused all the time? I don't like the way I feel."

I had taken her to a geriatric doctor for another opinion and unfortunately, he confirmed the dreaded disease.

"Mom, you have Alzheimer's." I answered quickly, not wanting to dwell on the subject.

"Thanks, thanks a lot. Crazy people get that disease." She said frankly, upset with the truthfulness I had just told her. I changed the subject and she quickly forgot what we were talking about. I never brought it up again.

The cold of winter and the cool of spring came and went with instances repeating themselves. It was now summer and again I came home for lunch as usual after she returned from the Center. The house was empty. The TV on, her pocketbook on the table and she was nowhere in sight. Panic set in. None of our neighbors were home and Mom was missing.

I called my son, who came home on his bike, and asked him to go around the block heading north; I'd head south, and we should meet where we find her in the middle. We met, but neither of us had seen her and the panic within me elevated. He went up another block and I went down the other; no Mom.

She had always told me that when she walked around the block that she would follow the concrete sidewalk and would always end up where she began; she usually did, but not today.

I said a quick prayer and asked God to help me find her safe and sound. With that, I heard several birds chirping in the playground across the street and there sat Mom on a bench under a tree whistling to the birds. I was never so happy to see her, but at the same time, I was furious that she had left the tranquility of the sidewalk. I tried to explain why we were so upset, but unfortunately, she just didn't understand our worry.

The next occurrence came when I arrived home from work another day for lunch and found all the windows open on a cool day at the beginning of October. The pungent burnt odor hit my nostrils as I walked up the front steps which caused me to race into the house.

Mom sat watching the TV, as usual, acting as nothing was wrong. The problem was she felt that nothing was wrong. Upon entering the kitchen, I couldn't help but notice a small saucepan filled with soapy water sitting in the sink. The bottom of the pan displayed the remnants of cooked coffee.

Oh, I thought, how many times did I tell her to heat up her coffee cup in the microwave—it was safer. But she continued to choose to pour cold coffee into a small saucepan and turn on the gas range. The soap never budged the burnt substance and I knew the problem was now beyond control.

I can't quite remember what was said that started the full force argument. My main worry was that she would seriously hurt herself and unknowingly start a fire. She, if only for a brief moment, realized there was a real problem and came out with the most surprising statement that was totally unexpected.

"Why don't you put me in one of those places where people like me live? It might be safer for everyone."

I had never thought of it. I guess I thought she'd never go along with a suggestion like that, but now that she had said it, the plan was set into action. We spoke about it for a couple days off and on. I didn't want to bring it up too much; I didn't want her to think it was my idea.

One Saturday afternoon she finally asked if there were any places nearby as she thought she'd like to go visit one. That's all the suggestion I needed. A new facility recently opened about one-half hour away and that was close enough for me to visit often.

The response to their visiting hours made me feel very comfortable with the place already. There were no set visiting times; people can come to see the facility whenever they wanted, morning, afternoon and early evening. She fell in love with the place immediately.

I had found out that Mom and Dad had purchased long-term care insurance which was the best thing she ever could have done. It was a three-year policy and would cover everything they had to offer.

Fake fireplaces, a library, a restaurant-styled dining room, several sitting rooms that looked like living rooms and tons of toys— dementia and Alzheimer's patients were going back in time and loved playing with toys in their second childhood.

She said she liked the facility and wanted to know if she could move here as she had already begun speaking with some of the residents. They had an opening, the paperwork was prepared, and she moved in at the end of the week.

I thought my life was about to go back to normal. We went through several seasons and Mom was enjoying herself and I was having the time of my life. We had two grandsons, whom Mom adored, and was so proud that she had become a great-grandmother. Unfortunately, her conversations always ended up with the fact that my father had missed these opportunities of seeing two young beautiful grandsons grow up.

With her mind still able to conduct a sensible conversation, she brought up her future, not once, but numerous times to make arrangements. She wanted to be donated for science and for someone to look at her brain and figure out how to stop Alzheimer's, for someone to have the ability to learn about the human body. She always wondered how surgeons could learn to properly operate on a person if they had to practice on a rubber dummy. I honored her wishes and the paperwork was filed with ***Humanity Gift Registry*** out of Philadelphia, Pa. Future doctors, nurses, and dentists would receive the gift of my mother when the time would arise.

As time passed, so did her mind. She was moved from an assisted-living area to the main dementia suite. It surprised me to see the number of residents; they weren't called patients in this section. How sad. A beautiful area, but it was a lock-down unit, only accessible by the means of a key coded elevator. Residents would walk past you, some with blank stares, some with full smiles, but emptiness behind them.

We would sit with Mom either in a living room or on warm days out on an enclosed patio shielded by a gazebo roof. She still enjoyed the warm air, maybe a fragment of memory from living in Florida.

Residents in the unit would see a trinket or gift lying around and think it was theirs and take them, so gifts to her had to remain generic and inexpensive—something that would be easy to replace. As her mind regressed backward, the obvious second childhood was pronounced. Dolls and carriages, vintage dresses and suits hanging on old-style clothes racks throughout the unit displayed the times that were. These were the times that were being remembered by those who lived here. It wasn't odd to see women carrying around baby dolls and stuffed animals; caressing them as if some were real and talking to them in adolescent voices.

My grandsons were surprised when we would buy children's toys and gifts for Mom. They didn't understand but enjoyed playing with the toys with Mom when we visited.

She was beginning to forget a lot more, and there wasn't that much left to forget. She had been married to my father for over 50 years and now she would look at his picture and think it was her brother who passed away 15 years ago. When I realized that she didn't know her husband, I wondered how long it would be before she didn't remember me. I thought that if I kept talking about daddy and kept repeating things to her, her mind would remember the love of her life. It didn't, and this only hurt me more. I wanted more than anything for her to remember her husband, my father. This state in her mind lasted for about another year. Then my world fell apart.

It was the day before Easter. I showed up for my visit with stuffed bunnies in hand and Mom had just finished lunch. One of the nurses in attendance said Mom was doing fine, but there had been a change and that I should be prepared. I escorted her to the sitting area to give her the Easter presents. She was full of smiles. Her head tilted back and forth as she hummed an old tune.

I handed her the unwrapped gifts as I kissed her and said hello. She looked up at me, caressing a yellow bunny, and with her big bright eyes said something that took my insides and twisted them. "Oh, how nice. Thank you." She lifted the bunny up under her chin and rubbed it back and forth. Then she turned her face to the side a little and dropped the bomb.

The words she uttered caused pain to soar through my heart. I had to catch my breath. "Are you a relation?" The words squeaked out of her mouth as if she was looking for the answer to a secret.

Sitting there in the chair, a young child's smile upon her face, eyes glowing like a child on Christmas morning, she looked at me. She looked right through me; only saw the appearance of a nice lady coming to visit. Not realizing that the person standing before her was her one and only daughter. I had to keep the fixed smile plastered on my face so she wouldn't see the hurt that consumed me. I shivered with the thought that mentally, my mother just lost me. I was no one she knew, a stranger, a nice lady.

It felt as if someone had reached inside me and ripped everything out. A pain I've never felt before. Even the death of my father didn't hurt this much. Standing before my mother, her only child, and she had no idea of who I was. I blinked back the tears that were fighting to be released. I knew I loved the woman facing me as my mother, but I also knew that if she still loved me, it was only as an unknown person.

"Yes." I whispered trying to force a smile so that she wouldn't see the hurt within me. She kept caressing the stuffed animals and began rocking back and forth as if to put an infant to sleep. The nurse walked in and realized that I had just learned the change in Mom.

"Are you all right?" Her voice indicated an understanding segment. "I'll be fine." My reply was a lie, I'm sure she recognized that.

"I'm sorry, it's something that I see much too often here in this unit. If it is any comfort to you, some of our residents get nasty at this stage. But your mother is a doll and is always smiling; I've never seen her in anything but a happy state. You should be thankful for that. It hurts the family members when their parents turn nasty."

It continued like this for an indefinite amount of time. Her long-term care insurance was running out and she had to be moved to `another facility. How I hate using that word, but it was the truth. Mom had issues and needed to be taken care of by people who fully understand deleterious affliction.

5

Since we had moved out of the area, Mom was moved to a facility closer to our home. Unfortunately, this time, it was a nursing home. I was petrified but the care there was wonderful. Each patient was treated as a family member. No matter when we went to visit, the warmth from the staff was evident.

The floor where she lived was a giant circle, but still a lock-down unit. The patients that could walk without assistance would walk non-stop; always ending up where they began, but never realizing it.

Mom always enjoyed helping others. Even with her mind habitually gone, she always was there to lend a hand. The nurses commented on how they appreciated her help. She would push some of the wheelchair-bound patients around and around the circle daily, freeing up their time to assist the needier patients.

The sad part was that the residents had to wear alarm warning bracelets. If anyone approached one of the exits in too close a proximity, an alarm would sound causing a nurse to calmly turn them around, and head them in a different direction. Some of the residents actually liked the alarm sound as their actions were displayed by pointing their fingers in the air, smiles on their faces, and emitting oh-oh sounds as if their fingers were dancing to the music.

It was evident that Mom's regression was increasing rapidly. Her good-mannered nature at times began to show nastiness. A trait I've never really seen in her. The nurses reported that there had been some issues with her not cooperating with them and being downright indignant. I soon learned it was a level of her that I detested.

I could, however, raise her spirits with the loved stuffed animals or baby dolls I would bring. I soon learned that I had to bring such items to each visit as they would disappear, being removed by other patients believing they were their gifts.

Several months had passed, and I was dealing with Mom's moods at times, which no longer changed upon my visit. She would point at one patient, then another and say nasty things and make faces; a side of my mother I quickly put out of my mind. I had to remember, this was not her, this was someone else. Unfortunately, this was someone I didn't like.

On a beautiful spring day, I decided to leave work a little early to visit Mom. But leaving work turned out to be earlier than I planned. The phone rang displaying the phone number of the nursing home.

"Mrs. Smith, we're calling you to let you know that we're having your mother transported to the hospital as something isn't quite right with her."

I left work and actually arrived at the hospital before she did. What I saw before me was totally unexpected. Mom's pale face and fixed gaze on the sky looked almost lifeless. She had no knowledge of anything or anyone around her.

IV lines were dripping into her arm, an oxygen tube was placed at her nose and monitors were beeping and displaying movements as blood pressures were taken randomly. The beeping echoed in my head. She was lying there, in an obvious semi-conscious state oblivious to her surroundings.

A staph infection was being fought off with the push of heavy antibiotics. Treatment had begun before informing me of the situation. I stared at her with tear-filled eyes. If treatment hadn't begun, she would have passed quickly seeing the condition she was in. I looked at the doctor. He apologized when I informed him that she had a DNR (do not resuscitate) Order and an order to withhold medications if there was going to be a non-reversal of a medical condition she may be experiencing. The nursing home didn't pass on that information—much to my dismay.

The nurses in the hospital displayed above average care for Mom. I took time off work and sat with her for several hours a day. Her now empty, apathetic eyes would glance at me from time to time. Only moaning sounds would come from her throat. All speech was absent along with the senility that remained.

Despite Mom's inability to communicate or anything else, she displayed the only natural response I would expect from her. She pulled the IV lines from her arms and fought off every attempt to insert a feeding tube. She couldn't swallow. It was their last resort for nourishment. She was sending me a message. She always told me she never wanted to be kept alive with tubes.

At the end of the week, I was informed that she had to be taken back to the nursing home as the hospital, at that time, didn't have a hospice unit. I knew the end was near. The nursing home had something called comfort care which was about to prove to me to be the most uplifting care I'd ever seen.

Mom was transported via ambulance and within two hours she was back in her bed. The soft, beautiful, relaxing music coming from the CD player next to her comforted us both as I entered her room. Curtains had been pulled around the bed to give her privacy, she had been placed in a clean gown and her hair had been combed. Her hands were soft as silk as I picked them up to caress them. I was informed that once an hour, she would be turned to avoid bed sores, and lotion would be softly rubbed onto her skin. She rested comfortably and was given pain medication every two to three hours.

It only took three days. Her comfort care was started on Friday and I received the call at 8 AM on a sunny Sunday morning. We sat with her for a long time. I still couldn't believe how soft her hands were from all the lotion. I knew this would be the last time I would see her as the arrangements were set for *Humanity Gift Registry* to pick her up tomorrow. The next time I would hold my mother, would be the day that I came to pick up her ashes when the fulfillment of her wishes after death had been completed.

I received notification that she had been picked up and delivered. I was thanked and would now have to wait at least a year before seeing her again.

****

The Memorial Service invitation arrived a year later. The auditorium at the school of medicine was large enough to hold the hundreds of family members in attendance. Soothing songs were sung by medical students and several key students, along with the Director of Humanity Gift Registry who gave compelling emotional speeches. The names of all those donated for the cause were listed alphabetically on the back of the program and it concluded with a light fare. It was emotional and uplifting at the same time. One more step forward for Mom, however, I knew it could still be up to one more year before I would bring her home.

Six months later the phone call arrived. It was time to pick up my mother. I was greeted with sincere thanks for the gift of my mother and was handed a cardboard box in a yellow handled bag after signing numerous documents. Mom was finally coming home.

The ride home was quiet. We drove as Mom sat on my lap and I couldn't help but reflect back on her unfortunate journey to this point. Had anyone learned anything from her brain or her body? Had her donation caused some kind of breakthrough in medicine? I'll never know, but I can pray that her donation wasn't in vain.

Now her ashes sit atop my bureau along with my father's, and I say good-morning and good-night to both of them every day. When it comes time for my burial, my parents will be buried with me, in my coffin—a suitable ending for their only child.

I miss them both, but mostly her, as I can't imagine what it's like to finish out your life forgetting everything about it and everyone you ever knew.

****

Having a parent, or loved one, go through Alzheimer's is devastating. It causes you to go through two grieving periods—one when you mentally lose the person, and one when you physically lose them. The first is more painful than the second. I lost mom's soul first. I lost the shell of her, second. Watching someone die twice is one of the hardest emotions I feel I will ever live through.

My prayer is that Alzheimer's and other diseases are cured and that our future doctors receive the highest level of education possible and that anyone reading this will consider **Humanity Gift Registry**. An organization devoted to medical education and research throughout the state of Pennsylvania with three locations.

The End

www.ingramcontent.com/pod-product-compliance
Lightning Source LLC
Chambersburg PA
CBHW070048260726

48658CB00002B/794